THE KIDNEY TRANSPLANT SMOOTHIES RECIPE BOOK

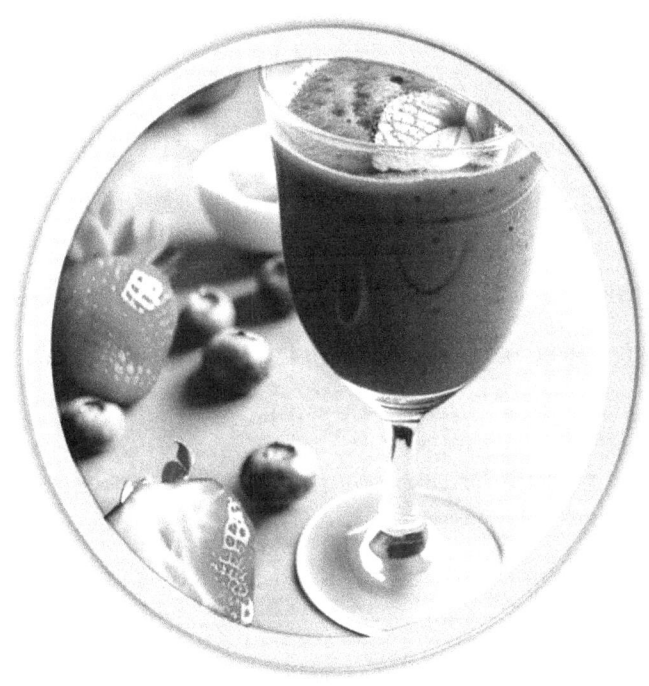

Empowering Your Recovery with
Tasty Smoothie Creations

Dr. Sarah Alber

Copyright © 2024 by Dr. Sarah Alber

All Rights Reserved

This literary work is protected by copyright laws and is provided solely for the private use of the original owner.

Unauthorized copying, adaptation, distribution, public performance, or other use of this work is strictly prohibited and may result in civil or criminal penalties.

Table of Contents

Introduction 8

The Importance of Smoothies in Kidney Health 11

Nutritional Guidelines for Kidney Transplant Recipients 17

Tips for Creating Kidney-Friendly Smoothies 24

Chapter 1: Breakfast Smoothies 31

1. Green Power Smoothie.................. 31

2. Berry Banana Bliss Smoothie 32

3. Tropical Mango Spinach Smoothie... 33

4. Creamy Avocado and Almond Smoothie... 34

5. Oatmeal Berry Breakfast Smoothie . 36

6. Pineapple Coconut Smoothie 37

7. Chia Seed Pudding Smoothie 38

8. Apple Cinnamon Oat Smoothie 39

9. Strawberry Almond Butter Smoothie 40

10. Peanut Butter Banana Protein Smoothie 41

Chapter 2: Refreshing Fruit Smoothies 43

1. Watermelon Mint Cooler 43

2. Peach and Ginger Smoothie 44

3. Citrus Sunshine Smoothie 45

4. Blueberry Basil Bliss Smoothie 46

5. Kiwi Lime Refresher 48

6. Raspberry Lemonade Smoothie 49

7. Blackberry Coconut Smoothie 50

8. Pomegranate Paradise Smoothie 51

9. Cherry Limeade Smoothie 52

10. Tropical Fruit Medley Smoothie 53

Chapter 3: Vegetable-Packed Smoothies................................... 55

1. Spinach and Cucumber Detox Smoothie.. 55

2. Carrot Ginger Energizer................. 56

3. Beet Berry Blast Smoothie 57

4. Kale and Pineapple Smoothie 59

5. Sweet Potato and Apple Smoothie... 60

6. Tomato Basil Smoothie 61

7. Zucchini Mint Smoothie 62

8. Avocado and Celery Smoothie 64

9. Green Goddess Smoothie 65

10. Roasted Red Pepper and Cucumber Smoothie.. 66

Chapter 4: Protein-Rich Smoothies 68

1. Almond Milk and Protein Powder Smoothie... 68

2. Greek Yogurt and Berry Smoothie... 69

3. Silken Tofu Chocolate Banana Smoothie... 71

4. Hemp Seed and Spinach Smoothie.. 72

5. Quinoa and Mango Protein Smoothie 73

6. Nut Butter and Oat Smoothie 75

7. Cottage Cheese and Pineapple Smoothie... 76

8. Edamame and Berry Smoothie 77

9. Chia Seed Protein Smoothie........... 79

10. Sunflower Seed and Banana Smoothie... 80

Chapter 5: Smoothies for Special Occasions 82

1. Holiday Spice Smoothie................. 82

2. Chocolate Mint Delight Smoothie 83

3. Festive Berry Medley Smoothie....... 85

4. Tropical Punch Smoothie 86

5. Matcha Green Tea Smoothie 87

6. Decadent Cocoa and Hazelnut Smoothie... 88

7. Caramel Apple Smoothie 90

8. Lavender Lemonade Smoothie 91

9. Gingerbread Smoothie 92

Conclusion 94

Introduction

Embarking on the journey of life after a kidney transplant is a significant milestone, filled with hope and new possibilities. As you adapt to your new lifestyle, nutrition plays a vital role in your recovery and long-term health. One of the most effective and enjoyable ways to incorporate essential nutrients into your diet is through smoothies.

The Kidney Transplant Smoothies Recipe Book is designed to provide you with a diverse collection of delicious, kidney-friendly smoothie recipes that cater specifically to your dietary needs. Each smoothie is carefully crafted to balance essential nutrients, ensuring you receive the nourishment required to support your new kidney while delighting your taste buds.

Smoothies offer a fantastic opportunity to combine fruits, vegetables, and protein sources into a single, easy-to-consume beverage. They are not only a convenient way to increase your intake of vitamins and minerals but also allow for creativity in the kitchen. Whether you're looking for a refreshing breakfast option, a quick snack, or a post-workout boost, this book has you covered.

In addition to providing a variety of smoothie recipes, we will also share tips on selecting the right ingredients, customizing flavors, and optimizing nutrition for your specific needs. You will learn how to create smoothies that are low in sodium, potassium, and phosphorus while still being flavorful and satisfying.

As you embark on this culinary journey, remember that your health is a priority. Embrace the flavors, textures, and nutrients in these smoothies, and allow them to be a vital part of your recovery. May this cookbook inspire you to explore new tastes and enhance your well-being as you embrace life after transplant.

Cheers to your health and happiness! Enjoy blending your way to a vibrant and nourishing future.

The Importance of Smoothies in Kidney Health

Smoothies have emerged as a popular choice for health-conscious individuals, and their role in kidney health, especially for those navigating life after a transplant, cannot be overstated. Packed with nutrients, easy to digest, and versatile in flavor, smoothies provide a convenient way to incorporate essential vitamins and minerals into your diet.

Here's why smoothies are important for kidney health:

1. Nutrient Density

Smoothies can be loaded with a variety of nutrient-rich ingredients, including fruits, vegetables, seeds, and protein sources.

This density allows you to obtain a wide range of vitamins, minerals, and antioxidants in a single serving, which is particularly beneficial for supporting kidney function and overall health.

Nutrient-dense smoothies can help bridge the gap when appetite is low, ensuring you still receive necessary nutrients.

2. Hydration

Proper hydration is crucial for kidney health, and smoothies can contribute significantly to your fluid intake. By using water, coconut water, or low-sodium broths as a base, you can create refreshing blends that help keep you hydrated. Staying well-hydrated aids in flushing out toxins and maintaining optimal kidney function, which is especially important post-transplant.

3. Digestive Ease

For many individuals recovering from surgery, solid foods may be harder to digest. Smoothies provide a gentle, easily digestible option that allows your body to absorb nutrients more efficiently. The blending process breaks down the fiber in fruits and vegetables, making it simpler for the digestive system to process and absorb the essential nutrients.

4. Customization and Control

One of the greatest advantages of smoothies is their versatility. You can customize them to suit your specific dietary restrictions and preferences. By carefully selecting ingredients, you can create smoothies that are low in sodium, potassium, and phosphorus while still being delicious. This level of control is essential for kidney transplant recipients who need to manage their intake of these nutrients to avoid complications.

5. Boosting Energy Levels

Smoothies can be a fantastic source of energy, especially when you incorporate healthy carbohydrates, protein, and fats. Ingredients such as bananas, oats, nut butters, and yogurt can provide sustained energy, helping you feel more active and engaged throughout the day. This is particularly important during the recovery phase when your body requires additional energy to heal and adapt.

6. Supporting Immune Function

The immune system plays a critical role in post-transplant recovery, and nutrition significantly impacts its function. Smoothies filled with fruits high in antioxidants, such as berries and citrus, can help strengthen the immune response. Additionally, incorporating ingredients like spinach or kale can provide essential vitamins, such as vitamin C and iron, which support overall immune health.

7. Encouraging Healthy Habits

Incorporating smoothies into your daily routine can foster a greater interest in healthy eating and cooking. Experimenting with different ingredients and flavors can help you discover new foods and encourage a diverse diet rich in fruits and vegetables. This shift toward healthier eating habits can contribute to improved long-term health outcomes.

Nutritional Guidelines for Kidney Transplant Recipients

Nutritional Guidelines for Kidney Transplant Recipients

Nutrition plays a pivotal role in the recovery and overall health of kidney transplant recipients. After a transplant, maintaining a balanced diet is essential for supporting the healing process, ensuring proper organ function, and preventing complications. Here are key nutritional guidelines tailored for kidney transplant recipients:

1. Focus on a Balanced Diet

A well-rounded diet should include a variety of foods from all food groups, ensuring you receive essential nutrients needed for recovery. Emphasize:

Fruits and Vegetables: Plan for a colorful variety to maximize minerals, vitamins, and antioxidants. Fresh, frozen, or canned (without added salt) options are all good choices.

Whole Grains: Choose whole grains such as brown rice, quinoa, whole wheat bread, and oats to provide fiber, which is important for digestive health.

Protein Sources: Incorporate lean proteins, such as poultry, fish, eggs, tofu, legumes, and low-fat dairy. These foods support tissue repair and immune function.

2. Manage Sodium Intake

Sodium control is crucial for preventing high blood pressure and fluid retention, which can stress the new kidney. To manage sodium intake:

Limit Processed Foods: Processed and the packaged foods often contain higher levels of sodium. Opt for fresh or for frozen foods whenever possible.

Read Labels: When purchasing packaged foods, check the sodium content and aim for options with lower levels.

Use Herbs and Spices: Instead of salt, flavor your dishes with herbs, spices, lemon juice, or vinegar to enhance taste without adding sodium.

3. Monitor Potassium and Phosphorus

After a kidney transplant, some individuals may need to manage their intake of potassium and phosphorus to prevent imbalances. Consult with your healthcare provider for personalized guidance:

Potassium: Foods high in potassium include bananas, oranges, potatoes, and tomatoes. Depending on your levels, you may need to limit these foods.

Phosphorus: Dairy products, nuts, seeds, and certain meats can be high in phosphorus. Monitor your intake, especially if you have elevated phosphorus levels.

4. Ensure Adequate Fluid Intake

Hydration is vital for kidney function and overall health. Aim to drink plenty of fluids, and primarily water, throughout the day. Depending on your medical team's recommendations, you may need to adjust your fluid intake based on factors such as:

Medications: Some immunosuppressive medications can affect hydration needs.

Physical Activity: Increased activity levels may require additional fluid intake to maintain hydration.

5. Prioritize Healthy Fats

Incorporate healthy fats into your diet, which can provide energy and support heart health:

Healthy Sources: Focus on sources of unsaturated fats, such as avocados, nuts, seeds, and olive oil. Limit saturated and trans fats intake found in fried foods and in many processed snacks.

Balance Omega-3 Fatty Acids: Consider including omega-3-rich foods, such as fatty fish (e.g., salmon, mackerel) and flaxseeds, which can support cardiovascular health.

6. Limit Sugar Intake

Managing sugar intake is important for maintaining a healthy weight and preventing diabetes, which can be a risk after a transplant due to certain medications:

Choose Natural Sweeteners: Opt for fruits to satisfy your sweet tooth instead of sugary snacks and beverages.

Watch for Added Sugars: Read food labels and avoid products high in added sugars, such as candies, pastries, and sugary drinks.

7. Consult with a Dietitian

Work closely with a registered dietitian who specializes in kidney nutrition. They can help you develop a personalized meal plan that meets your specific needs and preferences while ensuring you adhere to dietary restrictions.

Tips for Creating Kidney-Friendly Smoothies

Smoothies can be a delicious and nutritious way to support kidney health, especially for those recovering from a kidney transplant. However, it's important to ensure that the ingredients you choose are kidney-friendly and align with your dietary restrictions. Here are some practical tips for creating smoothies that are not only tasty but also beneficial for your kidney health:

1. Choose Low-Potassium Ingredients Wisely

While potassium is an essential nutrient, some individuals with kidney issues need to monitor their intake. Opt for fruits and vegetables which are lower in potassium, such as:

Fruits: Apples, berries (strawberries, blueberries), grapes, peaches, and pears.

Vegetables: Cucumbers, bell peppers, carrots, and leafy greens like spinach (in moderation).

2. Limit Sodium and Phosphorus

Avoid adding high-sodium ingredients to your smoothies, such as processed foods or condiments. Instead, enhance flavors with fresh herbs, spices, lemon juice, or vinegar. Be mindful of phosphorus levels as well; some protein sources, like nuts and dairy, can be high in phosphorus. Use them sparingly or opt for alternatives like almond milk (unsweetened) instead of cow's milk.

3. Incorporate Healthy Proteins

Adding a source of protein can make your smoothies more satisfying and beneficial for recovery. Opt for kidney-friendly protein sources such as:

Greek Yogurt: Look for low-fat or plain options.

Silken Tofu: Provides a creamy texture while being low in sodium and high in protein.

Protein Powder: Choose low-sodium, low-phosphorus protein powders that are specifically designed for kidney health.

4. Use Hydrating Bases

Start with a hydrating base for your smoothies to enhance flavor and increase fluid intake. Consider using:

Water: The simplest and most hydrating option.

Coconut Water: Naturally sweet and hydrating, but check potassium levels.

Herbal Tea: Brewed and cooled herbal teas can add flavor without sodium.

5. Add Healthy Fats in Moderation

Including healthy fats in your smoothies can help keep you full and provide essential nutrients. Consider adding:

Avocado: Offers creaminess and healthy fats while being low in potassium.

Flaxseeds or Chia Seeds: Both are high in omega-3 fatty acids and fiber, but use them in moderation to manage phosphorus levels.

6. Experiment with Flavor Combinations

Smoothies are an excellent canvas for creativity. Experiment with different flavor combinations so to keep things exciting. Some kidney-friendly combinations include:

Berry Blast: Blend strawberries, blueberries, and almond milk for a refreshing drink.

Tropical Escape: Combine pineapple, cucumber, and a splash of coconut water for a tropical vibe.

Green Refresh: Blend spinach, apple, and lemon for a nutrient-rich smoothie.

7. Be Mindful of Sugar Content

While natural sugars from fruits are generally healthy, it's still important to moderate sugar intake. Avoid adding sweeteners like honey or syrup, and instead rely on the natural sweetness of fruits. If you want a sweeter flavor, consider using frozen fruits, as they can enhance sweetness without added sugars.

8. Balance Fiber Intake

Including fiber in your smoothies can aid digestion and promote satiety. However, it's important to balance fiber intake, especially if you're new to a high-fiber diet. Start with small amounts of fibrous ingredients like oats, chia seeds, or leafy greens and adjust according to your body's response.

9. Plan Ahead and Prepare

Preparation is key to making healthy smoothies. Consider batch prepping smoothie ingredients by washing, cutting, and portioning them out ahead of time. Store them in the freezer for quick and easy access, allowing you to blend a smoothie in minutes.

Chapter 1: Breakfast Smoothies

1. Green Power Smoothie

Ingredients:

1 cup fresh spinach

1/2 banana

1/2 cup cucumber, chopped

1/2 cup unsweetened almond milk

1/2 cup ice

1 tablespoon chia seeds (optional)

Juice of 1/2 lemon

Preparation Instructions:

Add spinach, banana, cucumber, almond milk, ice, chia seeds (if using), and lemon juice to a blender.

Blend until smooth and creamy.

Pour into a glass and enjoy!

2. Berry Banana Bliss Smoothie

Ingredients:

1/2 cup frozen mixed berries. (blueberries, strawberries, raspberries)

1/2 banana

1/2 cup unsweetened almond milk

1 tablespoon honey or maple syrup. (optional)

1/2 cup ice

Preparation Instructions:

Place the frozen berries, banana, almond milk, honey (if using), and ice into a blender.

Blend until smooth.

Pour into a glass and enjoy!

3. Tropical Mango Spinach Smoothie

Ingredients:

1 cup fresh spinach

1/2 cup frozen mango chunks

1/2 banana

1/2 cup coconut water

1/2 cup ice

Preparation Instructions:

In a blender, combine spinach, mango, banana, coconut water, and ice.

Blend until smooth and creamy.

Serve immediately.

4. Creamy Avocado and Almond Smoothie

Ingredients:

1/2 ripe avocado

1/2 banana

1 cup unsweetened almond milk

1 tablespoon almond butter

1 tablespoon honey (optional)

1/2 cup ice

Preparation Instructions:

Add avocado, banana, almond milk, almond butter, honey (if using), and ice to a blender.

Blend until smooth and creamy.

Pour into a glass and enjoy!

5. Oatmeal Berry Breakfast Smoothie

Ingredients:

1/2 cup rolled oats

1/2 cup frozen mixed berries

1/2 banana

1 cup unsweetened almond milk

1 tablespoon honey (optional)

Preparation Instructions:

Combine oats, mixed berries, banana, almond milk, and honey (if using) in a blender.

Blend until smooth, allowing the oats to fully incorporate.

Serve immediately.

6. Pineapple Coconut Smoothie

Ingredients:

1 cup frozen pineapple chunks

1/2 banana

1 cup coconut milk (unsweetened)

1 tablespoon shredded coconut (optional)

1/2 cup ice

Preparation Instructions:

Place pineapple, banana, coconut milk, shredded coconut (if using), and ice into a blender.

Blend until smooth and creamy.

Enjoy!

7. Chia Seed Pudding Smoothie

Ingredients:

1/4 cup chia seeds

1 cup unsweetened almond milk

1/2 banana

1/2 cup frozen berries

1 tablespoon honey (optional)

Preparation Instructions:

In a bowl, combine your chia seeds and almond milk. Let sit for at least 30 minutes or overnight in the refrigerator until it thickens.

Once thickened, add the chia pudding, banana, frozen berries, and honey (if using) to a blender.

Blend until smooth.

Pour into a glass and enjoy!

8. Apple Cinnamon Oat Smoothie

Ingredients:

1/2 cup rolled oats

1 small apple, cored and chopped

1/2 banana

1 cup unsweetened almond milk

1/2 teaspoon cinnamon

1 tablespoon honey (optional)

Preparation Instructions:

Combine oats, apple, banana, almond milk, cinnamon, and honey (if using) in a blender.

Blend until smooth, making sure the oats are well incorporated.

Serve immediately.

9. Strawberry Almond Butter Smoothie

Ingredients:

1 cup fresh or frozen strawberries

1 tablespoon almond butter

1/2 banana

1 cup unsweetened almond milk

1/2 cup ice

Preparation Instructions:

Add strawberries, almond butter, banana, almond milk, and ice to a blender.

Blend until smooth and creamy.

Pour into a glass and enjoy!

10. Peanut Butter Banana Protein Smoothie

Ingredients:

1 banana

1 tablespoon natural peanut butter

1 cup unsweetened almond milk

1 scoop protein powder (optional)

1/2 cup ice

Preparation Instructions:

In a blender, combine banana, peanut butter, almond milk, protein powder (if using), and ice.

Blend until smooth and creamy.

Serve immediately.

Chapter 2: Refreshing Fruit Smoothies

1. Watermelon Mint Cooler

Ingredients:

2 cups seedless watermelon, cubed

1/4 cup fresh mint leaves

1 tablespoon lime juice

1/2 cup coconut water or regular water

Ice cubes (optional)

Preparation Instructions:

In a blender, combine the watermelon, mint leaves, lime juice, and coconut water.

Blend until smooth. If like, add ice cubes and blend it again for a cooler texture.

Pour into glasses and garnish with mint leaves. Serve immediately.

2. Peach and Ginger Smoothie

Ingredients:

2 ripe peaches, pitted and chopped

1 teaspoon fresh ginger, grated

1/2 cup Greek yogurt (or non-dairy yogurt)

1 cup unsweetened almond milk

1 tablespoon honey or maple syrup (optional)

Ice cubes

Preparation Instructions:

Combine the peaches, ginger, yogurt, almond milk, and honey (if using) in a blender.

Add a handful of ice cubes then blend until smooth and creamy.

Pour into glasses and enjoy!

3. Citrus Sunshine Smoothie

Ingredients:

1 orange, peeled and segmented

1/2 grapefruit, peeled and segmented

1/2 banana

1/2 cup unsweetened almond milk

1 tablespoon honey (optional)

Ice cubes

Preparation Instructions:

In a blender, combine the orange, grapefruit, banana, almond milk, and honey (if using).

Add ice cubes and blend until smooth.

Pour into glasses and serve immediately.

4. Blueberry Basil Bliss Smoothie

Ingredients:

1 cup fresh or frozen blueberries

1/4 cup fresh basil leaves

1/2 banana

1 cup unsweetened almond milk

1 tablespoon honey or maple syrup (optional)

Ice cubes

Preparation Instructions:

Add blueberries, basil leaves, banana, almond milk, and honey (if using) to a blender.

Blend until smooth, adding ice cubes for a chilled effect.

Pour into glasses and enjoy the refreshing taste!

5. Kiwi Lime Refresher

Ingredients:

2 ripe kiwis, peeled and chopped

1/2 banana

1 tablespoon lime juice

1 cup coconut water

Ice cubes

Preparation Instructions:

Combine kiwis, banana, lime juice, and coconut water in a blender.

Blend until smooth. Add ice cubes if you desired and blend again.

Pour into glasses and serve cold.

6. Raspberry Lemonade Smoothie

Ingredients:

1 cup fresh or frozen raspberries

1/2 cup lemonade (homemade or store-bought, low-sugar)

1/2 cup unsweetened almond milk

1 tablespoon honey or agave syrup (optional)

Ice cubes

Preparation Instructions:

In a blender, combine raspberries, lemonade, almond milk, and honey (if using).

Add ice cubes and blend until smooth.

Pour into glasses and enjoy!

7. Blackberry Coconut Smoothie

Ingredients:

1 cup fresh or frozen blackberries

1/2 banana

1 cup coconut milk (or almond milk)

1 tablespoon honey (optional)

Ice cubes

Preparation Instructions:

Combine blackberries, banana, coconut milk, and honey (if using) in a blender.

Blend until smooth. Add ice cubes for your chilled texture and blend again.

Pour into glasses and serve immediately.

8. Pomegranate Paradise Smoothie

Ingredients:

1 cup pomegranate seeds (arils)

1/2 banana

1/2 cup unsweetened almond milk

1 tablespoon honey (optional)

Ice cubes

Preparation Instructions:

In a blender, add pomegranate seeds, banana, almond milk, and honey (if using).

Blend until smooth, adding your ice cubes for a cooler texture.

Pour into glasses and enjoy!

9. Cherry Limeade Smoothie

Ingredients:

1 cup fresh or frozen cherries, pitted

1 tablespoon lime juice

1/2 cup unsweetened almond milk

1 tablespoon honey (optional)

Ice cubes

Preparation Instructions:

Combine cherries, lime juice, almond milk, and honey (if using) in a blender.

Add ice cubes and blend until smooth.

Pour into glasses and serve chilled.

10. Tropical Fruit Medley Smoothie

Ingredients:

1/2 cup pineapple chunks (fresh or frozen)

1/2 cup mango chunks (fresh or frozen)

1/2 banana

1 cup coconut water

Ice cubes

Preparation Instructions:

In a blender, combine pineapple, mango, banana, and coconut water.

Blend until smooth, adding ice cubes for a chilled effect.

Pour into glasses and enjoy the tropical flavors!

Chapter 3: Vegetable-Packed Smoothies

1. Spinach and Cucumber Detox Smoothie

Ingredients:

1 cup fresh spinach

1/2 cucumber, peeled and chopped

1/2 green apple, cored and chopped

1 tablespoon lemon juice

1 cup water or coconut water

Ice cubes (optional)

Preparation Instructions:

Combine spinach, cucumber, green apple, lemon juice, and water (or coconut water) in a blender.

Blend until smooth, adding ice cubes for a chilled texture if desired.

Pour into glass and enjoy your detox smoothie!

2. Carrot Ginger Energizer

Ingredients:

1 cup carrots, chopped

1 inch fresh ginger, peeled and grated

1/2 banana

1 cup orange juice

1/2 cup water

Ice cubes (optional)

Preparation Instructions:

In a blender, combine chopped carrots, ginger, banana, orange juice, and water.

Blend until smooth, adding your ice cubes if desired.

Pour into a glass and enjoy the energizing flavors!

3. Beet Berry Blast Smoothie

Ingredients:

1/2 cup cooked and peeled beets

1 cup mixed berries (fresh or frozen)

1/2 banana

1 cup unsweetened almond milk

1 tablespoon honey (optional)

Ice cubes

Preparation Instructions:

Place beets, mixed berries, banana, almond milk, and honey (if using) into a blender.

Blend until smooth, adding your ice cubes for a cooler texture.

Serve immediately and enjoy!

4. Kale and Pineapple Smoothie

Ingredients:

1 cup kale leaves, stems removed

1/2 cup fresh pineapple chunks

1/2 banana

1 cup coconut water

Ice cubes (optional)

Preparation Instructions:

Combine kale, pineapple, banana, and coconut water in a blender.

Blend until smooth, adding your ice cubes if desired.

Pour into glass and enjoy this tropical delight!

5. Sweet Potato and Apple Smoothie

Ingredients:

1/2 cup cooked sweet potato, mashed

1 apple, cored and chopped

1/2 teaspoon cinnamon

1 cup unsweetened almond milk

1 tablespoon honey (optional)

Ice cubes (optional)

Preparation Instructions:

In a blender, combine sweet potato, apple, cinnamon, almond milk, and honey (if using).

Blend until smooth, adding your ice cubes if desired.

Serve in a glass and enjoy!

6. Tomato Basil Smoothie

Ingredients:

1 cup cherry tomatoes, halved

1/4 cup fresh basil leaves

1/2 cucumber, peeled and chopped

1/2 cup unsweetened almond milk

1 tablespoon lemon juice

Salt and pepper to taste

Ice cubes (optional)

Preparation Instructions:

Combine cherry tomatoes, basil leaves, cucumber, almond milk, lemon juice, salt, and pepper in a blender.

Blend until smooth, adding ice cubes for a refreshing texture if desired.

Pour into a glass and enjoy!

7. Zucchini Mint Smoothie

Ingredients:

1 cup zucchini, chopped

1/4 cup fresh mint leaves

1/2 banana

1 cup coconut water

1 tablespoon lime juice

Ice cubes (optional)

Preparation Instructions:

In a blender, combine zucchini, mint leaves, banana, coconut water, and lime juice.

Blend until smooth, adding your ice cubes if desired.

Pour into a glass and enjoy the refreshing flavors!

8. Avocado and Celery Smoothie

Ingredients:

1/2 ripe avocado

1 cup celery, chopped

1/2 green apple, cored and chopped

1 cup unsweetened almond milk

Juice of 1/2 lemon

Ice cubes (optional)

Preparation Instructions:

Combine avocado, celery, apple, almond milk, and lemon juice in a blender.

Blend until smooth, adding your ice cubes if desired.

Pour into a glass and enjoy!

9. Green Goddess Smoothie

Ingredients:

1 cup fresh spinach

1/2 avocado

1/2 banana

1 cup coconut water

1 tablespoon lime juice

Ice cubes (optional)

Preparation Instructions:

In a blender, combine spinach, avocado, banana, coconut water, and lime juice.

Blend until smooth, adding ice cubes for a refreshing touch if desired.

Serve immediately in a glass.

10. Roasted Red Pepper and Cucumber Smoothie

Ingredients:

1 cup roasted red peppers (jarred or homemade)

1/2 cucumber, peeled and chopped

1/2 cup unsweetened almond milk

1 tablespoon lemon juice

Salt and pepper to taste

Ice cubes (optional)

Preparation Instructions:

Combine roasted red peppers, cucumber, almond milk, lemon juice, salt, and pepper in a blender.

Blend until smooth, adding ice cubes for a chilled effect if desired.

Pour into a glass and enjoy!

Chapter 4: Protein-Rich Smoothies

1. Almond Milk and Protein Powder Smoothie

Ingredients:

1 cup unsweetened almond milk

1 scoop protein powder (vanilla or chocolate)

1/2 banana

1 tablespoon almond butter

Ice cubes (optional)

Preparation Instructions:

In a blender, combine almond milk, protein powder, banana, and almond butter.

Blend until smooth, adding ice cubes for a cooler texture if desired.

Pour into glass to enjoy your protein-packed smoothie!

2. Greek Yogurt and Berry Smoothie

Ingredients:

1 cup Greek yogurt (plain or flavored)

1 cup mixed berries (fresh or frozen)

1 tablespoon honey or maple syrup (optional)

1/2 cup water or almond milk

Ice cubes (optional)

Preparation Instructions:

Combine Greek yogurt, mixed berries, honey (if using), and water or almond milk in a blender.

Blend until smooth, adding ice cubes for a chilled texture if desired.

Serve in a glass and enjoy!

3. Silken Tofu Chocolate Banana Smoothie

Ingredients:

1 cup silken tofu

1 ripe banana

2 tablespoons cocoa powder

1 tablespoon honey or maple syrup (optional)

1 cup almond milk

Ice cubes (optional)

Preparation Instructions:

In a blender, combine silken tofu, banana, cocoa powder, honey (if using), and almond milk.

Blend until smooth, adding ice cubes if desired for a cooler texture.

Pour into a glass and savor this creamy chocolate delight!

4. Hemp Seed and Spinach Smoothie

Ingredients:

1 cup fresh spinach

2 tablespoons hemp seeds

1/2 banana

1 cup unsweetened almond milk

1 tablespoon honey (optional)

Ice cubes (optional)

Preparation Instructions:

Combine spinach, hemp seeds, banana, almond milk, and honey (if using) in a blender.

Blend until smooth, adding ice cubes for a refreshing texture if desired.

Serve in a glass and enjoy the nutritious goodness!

5. Quinoa and Mango Protein Smoothie

Ingredients:

1/2 cup cooked quinoa

1 cup mango chunks (fresh or frozen)

1/2 banana

1 cup unsweetened almond milk

1 tablespoon honey (optional)

Ice cubes (optional)

Preparation Instructions:

In a blender, combine cooked quinoa, mango, banana, almond milk, and honey (if using).

Blend until smooth, adding your ice cubes if desired.

Pour into a glass and enjoy this protein-rich smoothie!

6. Nut Butter and Oat Smoothie

Ingredients:

1/2 cup rolled oats

2 tablespoons nut butter (peanut, almond, or cashew)

1 cup unsweetened almond milk

1 banana

1 tablespoon honey (optional)

Ice cubes (optional)

Preparation Instructions:

Combine rolled oats, nut butter, almond milk, banana, and honey (if using) in a blender.

Blend until smooth, adding ice cubes for a chilled texture if desired.

Serve in a glass and enjoy the hearty flavors!

7. Cottage Cheese and Pineapple Smoothie

Ingredients:

1 cup cottage cheese (low-fat or regular)

1 cup pineapple chunks (fresh or canned)

1/2 banana

1 cup unsweetened almond milk

Ice cubes (optional)

Preparation Instructions:

In a blender, combine cottage cheese, pineapple, banana, and almond milk.

Blend until smooth, adding ice cubes for a refreshing effect if desired.

Pour into a glass and enjoy this tropical smoothie!

8. Edamame and Berry Smoothie

Ingredients:

1/2 cup shelled edamame (cooked and cooled)

1 cup mixed berries (fresh or frozen)

1/2 banana

1 cup unsweetened almond milk

1 tablespoon honey (optional)

Ice cubes (optional)

Preparation Instructions:

In a blender, combine edamame, mixed berries, banana, almond milk, and honey (if using).

Blend until smooth, adding ice cubes for a chilled texture if desired.

Pour into a glass and enjoy!

9. Chia Seed Protein Smoothie

Ingredients:

1 tablespoon chia seeds

1 cup unsweetened almond milk

1/2 banana

1 cup spinach (optional)

1 tablespoon honey or maple syrup (optional)

Ice cubes (optional)

Preparation Instructions:

Combine chia seeds, almond milk, banana, spinach (if using), and honey (if using) in a blender.

Blend until smooth, adding ice cubes for a refreshing texture if desired.

Serve in a glass and enjoy this nutrient-rich smoothie!

10. Sunflower Seed and Banana Smoothie

Ingredients:

1/4 cup sunflower seed butter

1 ripe banana

1 cup unsweetened almond milk

1 tablespoon honey (optional)

Ice cubes (optional)

Preparation Instructions:

In a blender, combine sunflower seed butter, banana, almond milk, and honey (if using).

Blend until smooth, adding ice cubes for a chilled effect if desired.

Pour into a glass and enjoy this creamy, nutty smoothie!

Chapter 5: Smoothies for Special Occasions

1. Holiday Spice Smoothie

Ingredients:

1 banana

1/2 cup unsweetened almond milk

1/2 cup pumpkin puree

1/2 teaspoon cinnamon

1/4 teaspoon nutmeg

1 tablespoon maple syrup (optional)

Ice cubes (optional)

Preparation Instructions:

In a blender, combine banana, almond milk, pumpkin puree, cinnamon, nutmeg, and maple syrup (if using).

Blend until smooth, adding ice cubes for a cooler texture if desired.

Pour into a glass and enjoy the holiday flavors!

2. Chocolate Mint Delight Smoothie

Ingredients:

1 cup unsweetened almond milk

1 tablespoon cocoa powder

1/2 teaspoon peppermint extract

1 ripe banana

1 tablespoon honey or maple syrup (optional)

Ice cubes (optional)

Preparation Instructions:

In a blender, combine almond milk, cocoa powder, peppermint extract, banana, and honey (if using).

Blend until smooth, adding ice cubes for a refreshing texture if desired.

Serve in a glass and indulge in this chocolatey treat!

3. Festive Berry Medley Smoothie

Ingredients:

1 cup mixed berries (strawberries, blueberries, raspberries)

1/2 banana

1 cup unsweetened almond milk

1 tablespoon honey (optional)

Ice cubes (optional)

Preparation Instructions:

Combine mixed berries, banana, almond milk, and honey (if using) in a blender.

Blend until smooth, adding ice cubes for a chilled effect if desired.

Pour into a glass and enjoy the vibrant holiday colors!

4. Tropical Punch Smoothie

Ingredients:

1 cup pineapple chunks (fresh or frozen)

1/2 banana

1/2 cup mango chunks

1 cup coconut water

1 tablespoon lime juice

Ice cubes (optional)

Preparation Instructions:

In a blender, combine pineapple, banana, mango, coconut water, and lime juice.

Blend until smooth, adding ice cubes for a refreshing punch if desired.

Serve in a glass and enjoy a tropical escape!

5. Matcha Green Tea Smoothie

Ingredients:

1 teaspoon matcha green tea powder

1 banana

1 cup unsweetened almond milk

1 tablespoon honey or maple syrup (optional)

Ice cubes (optional)

Preparation Instructions:

In a blender, combine matcha powder, banana, almond milk, and honey (if using).

Blend until smooth, adding ice cubes for a refreshing touch if desired.

Pour into a glass and enjoy the energizing benefits of matcha!

6. Decadent Cocoa and Hazelnut Smoothie

Ingredients:

1 cup unsweetened almond milk

1 tablespoon cocoa powder

2 tablespoons hazelnut butter

1 banana

1 tablespoon honey or maple syrup (optional)

Ice cubes (optional)

Preparation Instructions:

Combine almond milk, cocoa powder, hazelnut butter, banana, and honey (if using) in a blender.

Blend until smooth, adding ice cubes for a chilled texture if desired.

Serve in a glass and indulge in this rich, chocolaty delight!

7. Caramel Apple Smoothie

Ingredients:

1 apple, cored and chopped

1/2 banana

1 cup unsweetened almond milk

1 tablespoon caramel sauce (optional)

1/2 teaspoon cinnamon

Ice cubes (optional)

Preparation Instructions:

In a blender, combine apple, banana, almond milk, caramel sauce (if using), and cinnamon.

Blend until smooth, adding ice cubes for a refreshing texture if desired.

Pour into a glass and enjoy the flavors of caramel and apple!

8. Lavender Lemonade Smoothie

Ingredients:

1/2 cup fresh lemonade (or lemon juice mixed with water)

1 tablespoon dried culinary lavender

1 banana

1 cup unsweetened almond milk

Ice cubes (optional)

Preparation Instructions:

In a blender, combine lemonade, lavender, banana, and almond milk.

Blend until smooth, adding ice cubes for a refreshing texture if desired.

Serve in a glass and enjoy this unique floral twist!

9. Gingerbread Smoothie

Ingredients:

1 banana

1 cup unsweetened almond milk

1/2 teaspoon ground ginger

1/2 teaspoon cinnamon

1/4 teaspoon nutmeg

1 tablespoon molasses

Ice cubes (optional)

Preparation Instructions:

In a blender, combine banana, almond milk, ginger, cinnamon, nutmeg, and molasses.

Blend until smooth, adding ice cubes for a chilled effect if desired.

Pour into a glass and savor the warm flavors of gingerbread!

Conclusion

As you close this chapter on your journey with smoothies, we hope you feel inspired and empowered to embrace a nourishing lifestyle post-transplant. The recipes in this book have been crafted with care to support your health, enhance your well-being, and introduce delightful flavors to your daily routine.

Smoothies offer a versatile and convenient way to incorporate essential nutrients into your diet. Whether you're seeking a quick breakfast, a refreshing snack, or a post-workout boost, these recipes provide you with a wealth of options to suit your taste and dietary needs. By focusing on fresh fruits, vegetables, and wholesome ingredients, you can create delicious blends that are not only enjoyable but also beneficial for your body.

Remember, the path to optimal health is a personal journey, and these smoothies are here to complement your unique nutritional requirements. As you explore the vibrant flavors and nourishing combinations, keep in mind the importance of hydration, balanced nutrients, and mindful eating. Your body deserves the best, and these smoothies are a step toward making your health a priority.

Thank you for joining us in this exploration of kidney-friendly smoothies. May your kitchen be filled with creativity and joy as you blend your way to better health. Cheers to your journey ahead—one delicious smoothie at a time!

www.ingramcontent.com/pod-product-compliance
Lightning Source LLC
Chambersburg PA
CBHW050328230526
45471CB00005B/2393